Leadership:

A List of Guiding Principles

Jeffrey Katz, MD

ISBN: 9798349469794

Dedication

All humans are destined to lead at some stage of their lives. This book is dedicated to all leaders.

Acknowledgement

This book was inspired by many mentors throughout my career who took the time to explain their decisions in challenging circumstances. The first leader who noticed me and took me under his wing was Joseph C. Gabel, MD, whom I met when I was recruited to the Department of Anesthesiology at the University of Texas in Houston. At that time, I had recently graduated from my residency in Anesthesiology at Mt. Sinai Hospital in New York, followed by my residency and fellowship at Case Western Reserve in Cleveland, Ohio. My fundamentals in leadership were laid down in that department in Houston. When I later became the Chair of that department, I continued to learn from a host of colleagues and leaders, too many to mention by name.

I would also like to thank Kathy Franz and her husband, Steven R. Patterson. Kathy worked as my right hand while I was Chair at UT Houston, and both she and her husband read my manuscript and offered many words of advice and wisdom. I also owe a debt of gratitude to my niece, Martine Savage, who read and commented on my content and offered insights based on her own extensive business experience. Chris Denman, RN, also reviewed the manuscript and encouraged me along the way.

I have been fortunate and honored to work with some of the most dedicated leaders, scientists, clinicians, and administrators during my career. Each has enriched the experiences and knowledge that went into this manuscript, and I deeply appreciate them all. I must single out Marco Evans and Hazel Quinn from Bestseller LLC, who have been remarkable in their dedication and hard work to make this book a reality.

Finally, I would like to thank my lifelong partner, Lesley, who, since the age of thirteen, has been my partner, teacher, friend, advisor, and chief supporter. Along with my three daughters, Cindy, Tracy, and Alexis, she has continued my education to this very day. Without all of these people, I would have had little to say, and no book would have been forthcoming.

One of my favorite phrases is, *"To be truly articulate, you must know when not to speak."* I know I have spoken enough.

Contents

Preface

Leadership is not a title, it is a responsibility, a calling, and often, a journey of trial and error. In every profession and at every stage of life, we find ourselves in situations where others look to us for guidance. Some rise naturally to the challenge; others hesitate, unsure of the principles or practices that define effective leadership. This book was written for both.

Throughout my career in medicine, administration, and education, I have observed leaders who inspired confidence, trust, and innovation, and others who struggled with basic, but critical, responsibilities. I was struck by how often errors in leadership stemmed not from lack of talent or intelligence, but from the absence of foundational guidance. Many colleagues would say, "Nobody ever told me that," revealing the gap between professional training and leadership preparation.

This book seeks to bridge that gap. It is not a textbook, nor is it meant to be a definitive authority. Rather, it is a collection of guiding principles, practical, tested, and refined through lived experience. Some lessons were passed to me by wise mentors who led with clarity and conviction. Others I learned the hard way, through mistakes, missteps, and the valuable reflections that followed.

The principles gathered here are universal. While my background is in healthcare, the challenges and opportunities of leadership are not confined to one industry. Whether you are leading a surgical team, a classroom, a business unit, or a community group, the values of trust, honesty, fairness, professionalism, and energy remain the same.

I invite you, the reader, not only to absorb these lessons but to engage with them. Make notes in the margins. Reflect on how they apply to your own journey. Challenge the ideas where you disagree, and expand on them where your experience provides new insight. My hope is that this book becomes less of a monologue and more of a dialogue, a living resource that grows richer as leaders at every level share their perspectives.

Ultimately, leadership is about people. It is about recognizing potential in others, nurturing it, and channeling it toward a mission greater than oneself. If this book helps even one leader act with greater clarity, humility, and courage, then its purpose will have been fulfilled.

— *Jeffrey Katz, MD*

Introduction

"If your actions inspire others to dream more, learn more, do more, and become more, you are a leader." John Quincy Adams

Throughout my career I have been fortunate to serve under remarkable leaders. Their mentorship and wisdom have greatly benefitted me, as they consistently took the time to share the reasoning behind their actions. This experience provided me with a well-rounded foundation that prepared me for my own journey as a leader and inspired in me a strong desire to pass on the valuable lessons I had gained. During my roles as a leader, I was often surprised to see that even those who had achieved considerable success in their careers sometimes made basic, avoidable errors or failed to carry out routine responsibilities. When I engaged them, I discovered that they had never been informed or taught about these basic steps and indeed spoke as if the education they had received as they progressed was almost non-existent. "Nobody ever told me that" was a common response. This project is an attempt to provide these basics to future leaders should they seek advice or council. Upon reviewing my educational background and preparation for senior leadership, I found that traditional education provided minimal direct training specifically aimed at equipping me for such roles. No text or written material was available to apply to specific challenges. Rather, I recalled many lessons learned by example, by *sub voce* advice, by critical conversations held after a meeting, or by observing my seniors manage a broad variety of challenges. Certainly, mentors played a pivotal role, and I recognized how lucky I had been to have been taught by exceptional teachers and insightful, experienced leaders, who instinctively knew the right course forward. I also learned that being truly articulate requires knowing when to stay silent and knowing how to respond effectively when necessary. So much meeting time is unnecessarily prolonged by participants feeling they were obligated to speak to preserve their perceived status within the group. Many leaders progress to leadership roles without being formally educated in leadership. Frequently, they are unable to attend college courses before they are assigned leadership responsibilities. Therefore, I present this booklet as a collection of my insights shaped by years of experience with the hope that I can fill in some of these gaps in education and stimulate thoughtful sharing of ideas from my readership in the form of a dialogue. These insights or skills can all be learned, or at least improved, if already present. Those who align with my ideas are encouraged to support them, perhaps with their own examples. Others who disagree are invited to share their own perspectives. My aspiration is that this publication will spark conversations about effective leadership preparation and impart wisdom in the conduct of leadership. Like all matters of conjecture, the more opinions expressed the richer the outcome of the discussion. Perhaps this booklet can evolve into a valuable resource for new leaders.

Therefore, I hereby invite both novice and seasoned readers to consider my ideas, and make notes as they read, so that once they are finished, their ideas can be submitted back to me for possible inclusion in an updated version.

Finally, it will be evident that my experience is founded in the healthcare industry, but I foresee that many of the issues I raise will apply to other situations in which leadership is key.

Description and Organization

The organization of the booklet is based on useful attributes I have identified over the years. Each is identified by a word or a phrase, which will be indicated at the beginning of each section. In each section, I have let my thoughts roam freely, sometimes giving examples of incidents I have experienced and other times working through a list of ideas. I expect that the material might jog a memory of an incident or experience that the reader has already encountered, that could either support my thoughts or stimulate a variety of contrary opinions which would add value to the script. If so, there is space at the end of each section that I hope the reader will use to note their thoughts for subsequent submission. The more ideas submitted, the richer the document will become. The number of sections is based on what came to mind as I wrote, so I expect there will be omissions, either because I did not remember them, or because they never occurred during my experience (i.e. I never learned that lesson). Once again, my hope is that if anything strikes the reader as missing or requiring correction or change, it should be noted at the end of the section and then submitted back to me using the mechanism described later.

In addition, there are some experiences which cannot be written in just a word or a phrase and contain good lessons. I plan to present those at the end of the booklet.

Most companies, institutions or organizations do not have one leader, they have a team. It is not necessary for every member of a leadership team to have all these attributes, or even most of them, to succeed. Indeed, I believe that fine leadership happens every day without many of them. But I also believe that knowledge of these attributes can help prepare the aspiring leader and provide guidance to workers who are new to leadership and might be quite intimidated. One of the earliest tasks a new senior leader (e.g. CEO) must approach is to build their own team, and one reason I am presenting this booklet is because I believe the characteristics I have included could be helpful to novice team members.

Leadership

"As we look ahead into the next century, leaders will be those who empower others." Bill Gates

There are many definitions and opinions of what the word leadership encompasses. It is not my intent nor is this the place to debate that question. Rather, I will present my ideas with the understanding that the extent and expectations of leadership can differ depending on where and when it is discussed. In this booklet, leaders are those who are responsible for an aspect of a company or entity's mission and can be the most senior in the company or a more junior person with limited responsibility. Either way, leaders are expected to provide guidance to those they lead and should have the skill and talent to influence others. Leaders should be motivated to identify the talents of their team members and be able to stimulate them to give their best to help advance the goals of the entity. Leaders should have the vision to foresee challenges and pitfalls and guide their employees away from missteps and stumbles. Leaders should understand the direction of their entity and should be willing to participate in strategizing and planning for future successes. Lastly, leaders should be models of professional behavior and, by example, guide their team members to a pathway towards advancing their goals. Despite the guidance given in this booklet, it is important to acknowledge that leaders are all human. Mistakes are part of doing your best, but new leaders should know that perfection is almost impossible to achieve. To act as if you are invulnerable would be arrogant and a mistake.

If I was asked to provide just three words of advice to leaders, they would be, Aim High, Trust your team members, and Adhere to your mission.

Understand How You Will Be Judged

"Not everything that can be counted counts, and not everything that counts can be counted." Albert Einstein

As a leader you should be judged on how well you advance the mission of your employer. As people assume leadership roles, they should make sure they thoroughly understand the expectations of the person who hires them. In business, this is usually going to be related to financial measures of success. This does not mean that aspects such as quality, efficiency or any other non-financial accomplishments are not important. But, even in an environment of excellent quality or efficiency an absence of financial success would be unlikely to result in a positive assessment. Similarly, average quality or efficiency with excellent financial gains are unlikely to lead to a negative evaluation. In business the mission is to make money.

In not-for-profit entities, there most likely will be goals such as quality, efficiency, beneficial impact etc. that are components of a performance evaluation and will be among the primary expectations of the employer. But it is important to remember that without financial viability it is unlikely that an entity will continue to make positive progress. Sister Generose Gervais, a founder of the Mayo Clinic, is noted for her quote "no money, no mission", and "no mission, no need for money". These lasting quotes underline the idea that financial resources should serve the mission, not be the sole objective.

Certainly, employers have a duty to provide expectations to their leaders, indicating with clarity where their priorities should land. But likewise, leaders must be clear on the expectations of their employers since without that clarity they are vulnerable to misdirecting their energies.

Aim High

"Shoot for the moon. Even if you miss, you'll land among the stars." Norman Vincent Peale and Les Brown

These words give a voice to the sentiment that encourages setting high goals and striving for greatness. The message here is that as a leader you will never be the best unless you aim for it. Many companies motivate their employees with a variety of messages to raise their ambition for reaching the top. But if the goal is for partial or incremental improvement, once you achieve that your job is not done, and you must raise your goals. Incremental success is not the same as accomplishing the best

Most industries rely on organizations or agencies to set standards in their fields. In many cases these standards are published annually in publications and top performers are identified. Achieving a top rating is an intensely motivating goal for the team members of an entity. Once accomplished, team members work intensively to sustain the rating. All in all, the goal of being the best is an important tool in the ongoing struggle to improve. There is no more crucial requirement than to constantly improve your mission.

Energy

"The world belongs to the energetic." Ralph Waldo Emerson

Of all the attributes that I shall cover, I believe ENERGY is perhaps the most important. Through the years, I have been most influenced by leaders who are able to appear energetic consistently, and radiate energy from the moment they are in your presence. They can sustain this energy despite stresses and setbacks and can, therefore, champion optimism and progress even when the odds appear to be against them. Most readers will remember people from their own experiences who brought this energy. They could have been teachers, religious leaders, or from any other walk of life in the past. Why is energy so fundamentally important? Because the most consistent challenge of leadership is the need to manage change. It is much more likely that a leader will be able to lead a team through change successfully if he introduces the need to change and a plan to make those changes with positive energy.

All of us have been in a meeting or gathering where the leader addressing the attendees seemed deflated, tired, unenthusiastic and frankly defeated. I clearly remember one such presentation during a strategic planning session, during which a colleague I respect texted me sarcastically with a one-word comment - "riveting!".

On the other hand, we also have been addressed by inspiring, positive leaders who have captured our attention as soon as they started speaking and kept us spellbound throughout their comments. This is the difference between having energy or not. Leaders who have energy are, among other things, consistently awe-inspiring, stunning, extraordinary and continually engaging. They elicit feelings of admiration, respect, and exceptional warmth and easily convince us of the merit of the points they are trying to make. In short, they are capable of exerting influence, one of the keys to successful leadership.

This expression of energy is not only evident in meetings or gatherings. It appears to emanate from them no matter where or when one is in their presence. They are forthright and look at people squarely in the eye. They make their case with such firm belief in what they are saying that people are on board before they complete their comments. They listen to responses with focused attention and stay in the moment while others offer their opinions. They are as energetic at the end of the day as they were at the beginning and seem able to continue for as long as it takes. Confidence radiates from them even while weighing challenging solutions, which might cause negative impacts on some established practices; but are required to effect changes that they believe are necessary. They remain creative and innovative no matter how jaded the audience might already be. They have the energy to keep people's minds present and engaged and are powerful enough to make others energized even when the prevailing environment might be unfavorable.

This energy might be confused with other positive attributes such as magnetism or courage, but at the end of the day, energy enables influence, and this is how leaders get others to respond and or follow.

Honesty

"Honesty is the cornerstone of all success, without which confidence and ability to perform shall cease to exist." Mary Kay Ash

HONESTY is a fundamental building block in sustaining a trusting environment. Furthermore, we also willingly embrace trust as a required aspect of excellent human interaction. Unfortunately, I have witnessed many walks of life in which participants have too easily changed their position on important issues without any explanation. To state the obvious, when one first meets a new colleague, team member or participant, it is reasonable to assume that they are honest, and indeed that sense would persist barring an experience where that honesty is breached. Honesty is therefore 'expected' and a reputation for honesty is easily granted. There is no need to prove it up front. But if it is ever surrendered by an act or assertion, it is instantly lost and becomes extremely hard to rescue. In healthcare, dishonesty can be life-threatening and the tolerance for dishonesty is zero. But in all walks of life, being dishonest, especially to protect oneself, is egregious and should be avoided at all costs.

Without trust, leaders cannot expect to deeply influence those whom they lead. Once the seed of doubt is planted, that doubt seems to encroach on an ever- increasing range of ideas being presented and undermines the quality of persuasiveness or influence that leaders must generate across the board. Once abandoned, trust is tantamount to impossible to re-acquire, and continued effective leadership becomes illusive. The minute a leader is known to have lied, his or her effectiveness in leading in the future is undermined, downgraded, and inevitably impaired. Honesty also implies transparency. Remember that attempting to be manipulative is dishonest and a dangerous gateway to loss of trust.

Sometimes, it becomes very challenging to sustain total honesty. You might hear something in confidence from a respected colleague which is potentially harmful to another close associate. You've promised to treat that information with discretion but have the welfare of your close associate in your hands. What do you do? Unfortunately, this is not unusual and might call upon your courage and judgement to manage wisely. In general, it is best to avoid getting into these types of conversations, but sometimes until the words are out, you cannot predict what will be said. Perhaps it is appropriate to advise your confidante to let your associate know what is being said ("you should tell him/her"), but sometimes that is not possible. Frequently, these situations will come back to haunt purveyors of gossip or rumor. (The truth always comes out). "If you're pleasing everyone, you're lying to someone" (Mike McDonnell. US Senator) is a phrase born out of bad experiences. Ultimately, simple as it sounds 'honesty is the best policy' (Benjamin Franklin)

Keeping Your Word (Deliver)

"If you break little promises, you'll break big ones." Cormac McCarthy; The Road.

Having already discussed 'Honesty', it might seem repetitive to approach keeping one's word in a separate section. But the two are subtly different. Dishonesty implies an intent to deceive. Failing to keep one's word frequently does not. Nevertheless, keeping one's word is of high importance and an area where leaders can easily fail and lose trust.

Sometimes, a leader accepts a position in which their success is directly linked to prevailing regulations, financial conditions or even promises. If those should change, it is possible that leaders might not be able to keep their word. It is not uncommon for conditions present at the time a leader begins their tenure to change according to fiscal, political, or other influences. Suddenly, a leader might find themselves unable to deliver on commitments made in good faith under different circumstances. How can leaders sustain their reputation of trustworthiness and reliability when this happens? Is it inevitable that trust will be lost? Not really, so long as these changes are clearly communicated and shared when they happen. I have seen leaders switch their position on a policy under their jurisdiction without explaining why. This is a recipe for loss of trust……they didn't keep their word.

Unfortunately, a loss of trust is also extremely likely to go viral rapidly. ("…. did you hear that our CEO flexed 180 degrees on our agreed process for……")? Once again, how big changes in conditions are communicated is of vital importance if trust is to be preserved. And the timeliness of this communication is key. Waiting until the change is publicly appreciated is too late. Team members will be understanding and forgiving if an explanation is provided early, and even more supportive if plans for recovery are shared or enlisted concurrently.

Keeping one's word is important both to employees and those senior to them, (one to whom you report), and junior (those who report to you). In the case of those to whom one reports, they will rapidly become doubtful of your ability if promises to complete tasks, deliver reports, meet deadlines etc. are not ready when you said they would be. This will directly impact on your reputation for reliability. Once people realize that you cannot deliver what is asked of you, they will cease to assign important tasks or projects to you. Loss of these tasks will rob you of opportunities to present new ideas and lead the direction of your team. They will also advise others that giving it to you would lead to a delay since you are unreliable. Finally, they will tell others that you are not reliable, and you will cease to function as a reputable team member.

Likewise, if one repeatedly does not keep their word with those that report to them, they will soon be viewed as unreliable, and subordinates will talk among themselves and spread the word. Eventually comments like "I wouldn't ask him or her, you'll never hear back" will become commonplace.

The importance of keeping your word should be understood and instinctive to individuals on the path to leadership, and yet, I have witnessed this important skill managed very poorly. People sometimes don't return calls and fail to reply to email messages because they have failed to complete their promised task. This rapidly leads to the kind of reputation I highlighted above. If a timeline appears too aggressive, it should be pointed out at the time the deadline is established rather than taking the liberty to deliver late.

It should be obvious that keeping to one's word is a desirable characteristic, and those on the road to advancing their careers will work to ensure that they do. Those that do not will languish, flounder, and progress will become challenging.

Change

"The only constant is change." Heraclitus (535–475 BC)

People resist CHANGE for many reasons, but leaders know that change is inevitable and that they will have to constantly manage it. Imagine how strongly you become wed to a change which is hard to do and took a long time to accomplish. You adjust, get used to it. But then guess what? You must change again. That is why people resist it. Humans are actually very good at adjusting to change. They rapidly become accustomed to the new conditions.

As a leader, you will have to embrace change like never before. You will have to decide to change; plan on what changes to make; communicate the reason and need to change; identify the changes to be made; lead the execution of the changes; monitor measures to evaluate the success of the changes; and prepare for the same cycle once again.

Why is this so? Change is required to respond to the need for constant improvement. All missions have goals, and usually there are mechanisms in place to measure progress towards those goals. In a successful entity even if you achieve your goals, there is a cultural mission to constantly do better. Measures monitor progress towards the goals and are regularly reset (changed) according to prevailing conditions (e.g. the market, competitive influences and the duty to keep improving.). In this sense, change is like growth; it must continue to progress, or the entity is failing. There are exceptions; for example, an entity can make a strategic decision to reduce activity in an aspect of their scope of business for a variety of reasons, especially if that activity has evolved to be less desirable than before.

An elegant example is the reduction in Coronary Artery Bypass surgery (extremely lucrative) because non-invasive therapies have arisen which achieve better results with less effort, complications, discomfort for the patient and cost. When coronary surgery was first discovered, it stimulated a huge change (and success) in the management of ischemic heart disease. That rapidly became the standard and behavior changed universally to improve clinical outcomes. Now, new knowledge has again stimulated change, and surgery for ischemic heart disease has become less common, as less invasive coronary artery stenting has grown. This will surely change again with new science.

To remain energized and enthusiastic about change is stressful for even the best of leaders. Leaders must be flexible and stubbornly persistent as they drive their teams to change. Leaders must infuse resilience and toughness into their team members, which focus on change as an ever-present challenge.

Trust

"He who does not trust enough will not be trusted." Lao Tsu (571 BC)

TRUST is established by being stringently honest and faithfully keeping one's word. It goes without saying that if your team can't trust you, your chances of being a successful leader are low. However, the mutuality of building trust is equally important. Leaders must be able to trust their team members. Once a team is appointed and assigned, leaders must trust the members unless there is reason not to.

Many readers of this publication will recognize the consequences of not trusting a team. Initially, as a leader, if you do not trust a team member you check on them repeatedly, and this is quickly sensed by the team member and other team members. This sparks questions among the team that others might not be trusted, and team members begin looking over their shoulders to see if they are trusted. Without a prompt explanation from the leader as to why they are checking up so frequently the team member loses confidence and becomes tentative and less effective. By being extra cautious he begins to weigh other team members down. If the leader threatens his membership on the team, a toxic cycle is set up with team members doubting their own safety on the team. An effective team requires the membership to feel free to openly express their support or opposition to plans being contemplated, and once doubts about individuals are raised, the team becomes less effective and ultimately fails.

New leaders are expected to decide on their team quite soon after their appointment. What if they are replacing a leader who had an effective team in place? Good employees are difficult to replace and if a team has worked successfully in the past, it is wise for a new leader to exercise patience, observe carefully how the team operates and analyze his own ability to work with those team members. If the new leader has a sense that he would be able to build trust in the team membership, it is perfectly acceptable, and sometimes preferable to keep the team in place and watch how performance unfolds. A working team will be more able to work with a new leader if they are informed up front that no changes are planned for a finite period, reserving the right to make changes later if necessary.

Team dynamics are occasionally complicated and challenging to manage. When a new leader is appointed, they are usually given the resources and support to build their own team. Employers know how important healthy team dynamics are and will have patience with new leaders as they sort out their requirements. For a new leader, failure to build a trusting relationship in both directions will undermine their chances of success. Although this is a less common conundrum for more junior leaders, even novices should understand the cruciality of trust in their team members.

Professionalism

'A professional is someone who can do his best work when he doesn't feel like it." Alistaire Cooke

When you become a leader there is a reasonable expectation that you have displayed the traits of a leader and indicated that you are able to influence other workers. As you rise in a company, there is also an expectation that your values, behavior, conduct, judgement and attitude will reach a higher level as you advance.

PROFESSIONALISM is achieved when the above characteristics are consistently in harmony with the high standards established by your company. Even if you believe you are professional, it is one of those things where there is no limit, and where continual improvement must be your goal. Professionalism means you do the right thing, say the right thing the right way, and experience very few lapses.

Professionalism includes a variety of components of performance, but most of them involve never crossing boundaries which have been established over years of experience. Etiquette is probably the aspect that is most often involved in lapses. Etiquette is about how you behave, interrelate, speak and treat other people. Personal boundaries are an important part of etiquette and are established to ensure personal privacy, discretion and safety. Employees in general should never initiate or pursue personal relationships involving employees, especially unwanted advances with workers who are junior to them in the company. Leaders should be fastidious about avoiding this. Despite this well recognized transgression, unwanted or unsought advances are frequently identified in lapses of professionalism in either gender. This is sometimes a difficult issue to manage since many individuals meet their spouses at work. If relationships naturally develop and grow at work, it is imperative that the couple exercise discretion or consider being open about it. Once other workers are aware that a relationship is present, they're immediately on watch for nepotism and favoritism. Other etiquette standards exclude the use of bad language, abusing other workers verbally, speaking negatively about other employees, or being contemptuous of co-workers, especially in public. Other aspects of professionalism include honesty, competence, respect, confidence, accountability, decency, civility, fairness and kindness. I will enlarge on these characteristics throughout this booklet which is presented to improve professionalism. But the main purpose of this booklet is to help you become a better leader. All workers must be as professional as they can. Any lapse in professionalism can seriously harm your efforts to become a better leader. Lapses in honesty, discretion and personal interactions are most likely to diminish your record of professionalism. Things like attire and timeliness can differ from company to company and it is imperative that as a leader you understand the standards at the institution where you work.

Honesty and discretion have been raised in other parts of this booklet. Competence is kind of obvious, since if you can't do the work, you should not be leading it. Are you able to keep your commitments, deliver on time, and perform as expected of a leader? Do you plan and strategize in an organized manner, and can you demonstrate a continual effort to improve your skills and learn? This is closely related to accountability since if you do make an error, it is very important to recognize it, own it and commit decisively to learn from it.

Respect refers to how you treat all the various groups of people with whom you interact. These include your bosses, your reports, your customers, and all employees no matter what their level. Respect manifests as being in the moment during conversations, paying close attention to what people are saying, and responding supportively and kindly. Respect includes empathy and sensitivity about other employees' challenges and aspirations. Respect does not equate with agreement with another, but acknowledgment of another's seniority. Respect also includes avoiding speaking about others negatively. It is disrespectful to talk over others or interrupt them while they're speaking.

Competence is about how well you do your job. Are you able to keep your commitments, deliver on time, and perform as expected of a leader? Do you plan and strategize in an organized manner, and can you demonstrate a continual effort to improve your skills and learn?

Confidence is measured by how sure you are of your ability to manage your business. Do you hesitate and second-guess yourself or do you present plans positively and with clarity? Are you realistic about what you can achieve, and do you seek help when indicated? Having an accurate sense of your own skill set is a part of professionalism. When you overestimate your own ability, you stray into arrogance, a sure way to degrade your professionalism and certainly a flag to others that you are not as good as you think you are.

Civility means that you pay complements when they are deserved, express sympathy when indicated and exhibit generosity of spirit when you can. Actual generosity is a personal decision but is still a part of civility, and a balanced approach to generosity is important. Similarly, having good manners is expected, especially not being rude to others, particularly those junior to yourself. It is uncivil and rude to talk while somebody else is already talking or during a presentation.

Being fair is an aspect of professionalism that is of particular interest to junior employees. It is important for leaders to be concerned about fairness and to focus on this when determining compensation, time off, schedules, and vacations. Having the perception that they are fair is an important goal for leaders.

Kindness is frequently forgotten by leaders, especially when under stress and struggling to get a grip on some nagging problem. Kindness should come naturally to leaders, and a lack of kindness will be felt, especially by younger or less mature employees. If you become aware that you were unkind either by being told or by suddenly realizing it, it is imperative that you immediately identify it and apologize as early as possible. People will tolerate a lack of kindness if an apology is rapidly expressed but will be hurt if not. This type of hurt is painful to workers and lasts much longer than expected.

Elsewhere, I mention the negative aspects of drifting into an 'in-group' scenario. A related area is allowing a punitive or toxic mindset to develop among your team. Toxicity arises when employees feel disrespected and subjected to bias, hurting their self-esteem and confidence at work. This very negative sense sometimes develops slowly and covertly. Just a couple of negative comments, sarcasm, disrespect, mocking or expressions of doubt can result in the deterioration of a previously good work environment. The subjects of such treatment will rapidly seek solace among others whom they perceive to have been objects of similar maltreatment, and a toxic cycle is set up. Similarly, if a misstep is harshly criticized in public, the same could happen. Leaders must always have their antennae raised and be very cautious about how they address team members. Quite frequently, toxic environments are only discovered when anonymous questionnaires about areas of dissatisfaction are circulated and respondents become willing to be candid because they cannot be identified. This is good evidence that a punitive cycle prevails and calls for swift remediation. In these situations, leaders are sometimes totally unaware, but on reflection, understand the origin and can, with sensitivity, humility and tact, reverse the negative spiral. Allowing this milieu to fester on would be unprofessional and damaging to a leader's reputation.

Confidence

"Believe you can and you're halfway there." Theodore Roosevelt

Having CONFIDENCE rates a separate section even though it also is part of the section on Energy. There is no doubting the attractiveness and magnetism of high confidence. There are also many very accomplished leaders who do not project confidence as an obvious characteristic. They might exude competence and dedication but maintain a slight tentativeness which comes across as modesty. Indeed, the charms of understatement and calmness often are preferred to exuberance and stardom. Nevertheless, it would be hard to project confidence without a good dose of energy.

If we recognize the importance of persuading and influencing others as a key role in leadership, then it is difficult to imagine a leader being able to convince others of his ideas without a reasonable measure of confidence in those ideas. I have experienced appropriate confidence, where the idea is obviously righteous and the function of leadership is easier; and tentativeness when getting others to follow is a struggle because the idea is possibly flawed, too novel or at least unsure in its outcome. Being tentative is not that uncommon because in any dynamic team, opinions vary, and there are frequently opposing ideas to those being advocated by a leader. In that scenario, confidence can be a useful tool in advancing an idea. History illustrates that leaders in many walks of life have persuaded their followers with doubtful evidence and great confidence and landed up leading them into a chasm.

Despite this, I still believe confidence is a good characteristic for leaders to have. If you already have it and you want to lead, it is a good thing. If you are not naturally so, gaining education, doing your homework, practicing your trade, and seeking council from those more knowledgeable than you are good exercises to raise your own level of confidence.

Conversely, over-confidence is a handicap. If people view you as over-confident, you have to find a way to assuage your exuberance or you might come across as arrogant. Industry is replete with arrogant leaders, and many of them have accomplished great success, so if that is where your advantage resides, it will be quite challenging to reverse that behavior. If you view yourself as comfortable in this mode of behavior, you hardly need advice to become more confident. Over confidence can also be interpreted as bullying, another trait which is unwelcome to workers.

Reliability and Safety

"Until we have established reliability there is no sense at all in wasting time trying to make things go faster." Carroll Smith

Whether you're manufacturing widgets, mining bitcoin, deep-sea fishing or fighting forest fires, the more RELIABLE you are in your processes the more success you will have. Conversely, if your systems are unreliable, success will be elusive, and your customers will know it. Likewise, the safety of your teams and employees, both physically and emotionally, should be prime goals for leadership. A moment's thought will lead you to understand that to keep employees safe, your systems must be reliable. As a new leader, some aspects of reliability and safety might appear to be slightly out of scope in conversations about traditional leadership, but experienced leaders will identify strongly with the sentiments expressed above. Even though systems and processes are the mechanisms by which work gets done, culture is where achieving high reliability resides.

In classical teaching about achieving high reliability there are five main principles which best describe the pathway to accomplishing it; an abiding preoccupation with failure, reluctance to simplify, sensitivity to operations, commitment to resilience and deference to expertise. Even though a leader cannot be expected to manage all of these every day, building a culture and recruiting a team is the leader's direct responsibility. Similarly, the leader is tasked with making sure that the safety of his employees is actively managed, and that the right managers are on site. Sensitivity to operations calls for at least one expert who understands the total operation of the entity and is tasked with keeping his finger on the pulse of the company. A reluctance to simplify ensures suitable attention to detail so that crucial details do not slip under the radar. A commitment to resilience demands a culture where teams return rapidly to highly reliable processes after an error or catastrophe occurs. Deference to expertise creates a culture where the expertise in the company is determined by experience and knowledge, not position. During trying times leaders are willing to go to junior workers on the line and seek advice if that is where the expertise exists. These are all under the direct authority and responsibility of the leader. Highly reliable entities are able to consistently carry out stressful tasks for long periods of time under challenging conditions.

While the safety of workers is most frequently assigned to human resource (HR) personnel, it is the responsibility of the leader to support HR regulations, laws and processes and to ensure that dignity, emotional support and fairness are sustained under his watch.

Communication

"Communication is the oil that lubricates the world's industries."

Volumes have been written about the importance of COMMUNICATION. Since this publication is a guide, a list of guiding ideas is featured below. Live communication is the most important language of leadership and should always be clear and easy to follow. Here are some items which should be followed by leaders no matter what their level in the company:

1. Live face-to-face conversation is always the best form of communication. There is no guarantee that emails and texts have been received or understood. Live conversation also allows an immediate observation of body language and how the conversation has been received. It is wise to follow up live interactions with written confirmation.

2. If you are responding to a communication or have something you need to say, do not delay. The sooner you communicate the better. On the other hand, if the subject for communication has induced an emotional response it is wise to delay since emotions have been known to stimulate comments which have been regretted later. If your message is urgent, you should indicate that clearly.

3. Communication starts with a greeting. Leaders should always open with a warm, friendly and upbeat greeting.
4. Communication always gets better when the dignity of participants is respected.
5. Whenever possible, an expression of gratitude to your team members is excellent practice. Certainly, when something is done to advance your mission, a thank you should be part of your communications.
6. When responding to emails, texts or letters, always read the full message and be fully responsive when you write back. It is frustrating to receive replies which fail to address items in the original inquiry.
7. When people come to talk to you, it is essential that you listen attentively, avoid being disturbed and refuse double-tasking and interruptions. Let your visitor have their full say. Be in the moment and remain there until you are both done. Sometimes senior participants in a conversation will use interruption and subtle subject change as a technique to disarm or intimidate the junior participant. This does not usually produce positive outcomes.
8. It is best to remember names and use them while looking directly at the person with whom you are speaking.

9. Never ignore a person who is trying to talk to you.
10. Whenever you can, smile, express warmth and be appropriately friendly.
11. When you are told something, you owe yourself a thorough investigation / confirmation of what has been said. Do not just take one opinion. Always check the facts, if possible. You should not form fixed opinions based on one person's assertions. Much harm has been brought by casual untrue comments thrown out during a conversation.
12. When communicating in a large space such as a meeting room and using slides for your presentation, make sure your slides will be legible at the extreme back of the space. Showing complicated small print information that is illegible is a waste of your time and that of your audience. If it is your intent to show a large complex process, show it on one slide first, but then break it down into smaller digestible slides while you explain.
13. If you are using a pointer do not wave it around the slide material rapidly. The audience cannot follow it and will not understand the points you are making. Furthermore, the further away the audience is from the slide, the worse fast pointer sweeps look.

14. Slides should be used to remind you of your next thought. You should know your material and be ready to speak fluently once you have been reminded by the slide. Reading your own slides verbatim is not a good style of presentation since the audience can always read it faster than you can announce it.

15. Assume that every conversation conducted in private is intended to be discrete. Do not leak personal or private information.

Presence

"We convince by our presence". Walt Whitman

It is tempting to rely on other team members to be visible and spend more time in your office planning and meeting. There are some very important advantages to gain by being out and about in your company.

The first is that the only way you can gain a thorough understanding of what life is like as a member of your team, is to be there. Apart from experiencing the actual physical environment e.g. the air conditioning doesn't work well, the noise level is very high, there is a light bulb that hums, etc., is to share in those experiences yourself. There is also the emotional ambience that workers on your team experience. Is there silence in the work area, or are your team members interacting, helping each other and feeling positive most of the time? This is relevant in any environment, a factory floor, an office, or even an outside area. When team members come to you to ask for a change, something new or a move perhaps, it will be meaningful to you. You will be able to picture their discomfort and respond with measures that approach their actual complaint.

Another reason to be out and about is to make sure your team members know that you are at their side supporting them most of the time. If workers are wondering what it is their supervisor does all day long, their trust in your leadership is already undermined. At times, it is necessary for you, as a leader, to have full privacy and be apart from your team, but this should always be mixed with spontaneous interludes of your presence, which reassures them that you are engaged and familiar with what they are doing.

The message given by a leader's presence at the work site is positive and supportive. A lack of visibility gives rise to doubts and questions.

Fairness

"A fair-minded person tries to see both sides of an argument."

Aesop

While preparing for this publication I had several opportunities to ask colleagues and friends what they thought was the most important aspect of leadership. Several successful people identified FAIRNESS as of primary importance. On deeper inquiry, these people cited issues over salary and time assignment as the reason fairness is so important to them. There are several interesting quotes on fairness that state that equal pay should not be a measure of fairness. Indeed, the idea that pay should be distributed more on performance and effort was more common. John Wooden (college coach) wrote that "Fairness is giving all people the treatment they earn and deserve. It doesn't mean treating everyone alike."

Yet, I am convinced that "protected time and pay" is the cause of a large measure of employee dissatisfaction with their leadership. Traditionally, pay is usually held as discrete information, whereas protected time (time to complete tasks of interest to the entity's mission, but outside the worker's direct job description) is frequently obvious to other workers and more likely to cause dissatisfaction. In state or government institutions the details of pay are frequently available to others upon request and privacy cannot be guaranteed.

Apart from the two above subjects above, other challenges to fairness exist in how differences of opinion are adjudicated, especially arguments among employees, which are better reviewed by human resources personnel than decided by leaders.

Nevertheless, fairness is clearly an area where leadership can be challenged, and leaders should be willing to seek assistance from impartial judges if possible.

Ideas

"The air of ideas is the only air worth breathing." Edith Wharton

The importance of new IDEAS is recognized and emphasized in almost all entities today. Generation of new ideas should be one of the most urgent tasks on the priorities list of modern leaders. Without new ideas, institutions are doomed to slow progress, stagnation or even decline. The burden for creativity and innovation weighs on the shoulders of leaders. Leaders must create an environment in which creativity is welcome, innovation is prized, and new ideas are championed. Leaders should regularly make time for discussion of new ideas and nurture an environment in which employees at every level are encouraged and rewarded for being creative. In my experience, there was little that was more stimulating than participating in an executive team where new ideas were discussed at every meeting regardless of their ultimate acceptance or rejection. New ideas should never be regarded as bad ideas; only ideas that might not fit the current circumstances or environment and should be preserved for consideration when prevailing conditions change.

Many entities have developed programs to stimulate the generation of new ideas. Such programs are usually offered to employees at every level. Many of these programs include rewards for innovative ideas that become adopted and communicate these ideas broadly and frequently to all employees. Companies in which ideas are considered valuable and appreciated are more likely to succeed and certainly are seen by their competitors as leading their industry.

The importance of seeking ideas from employees at all levels is fundamental to institutions that aim for high reliability. Employees doing the work of the company are very likely to recognize processes that are inefficient or wasteful. If these workers are omitted from the search for new ideas, valuable knowledge and experience will be left out of the equation. A fundamental principle of high reliability is paying deference to expertise. A considerable portion of expertise in any company resides in the working ranks, no matter how far they are from top management. It is inconceivable to expect that employees working in an office would know more about production inefficiency than those laboring on a production line. Entities that recognize and practice deference to expertise will have a more engaged workforce overall because workers feel acknowledged and valued when encouraged to give their opinion.

Leaders cannot treat innovation as one of those duties that will take care of itself. Without creativity and innovation, companies will be starved of oxygen. Dedication to creativity must be intentional and detailed and part of every leader's incentive. Creativity and innovation are linked very closely to research.

While pure scientific research is more the burden of educational entities, all industries should have their eyes on current research in their areas of operation. Curiosity should be encouraged and nurtured by all entities as the initiating force in improving themselves. The quest to improve all facets of an entity's activities is a fundamental aspect of advance, progress and success. From a leader's point of view, they should be constantly updating and upgrading their systems and processes and must rely on new discoveries and innovations to provide guidance as to what is next. It is therefore incumbent on leaders to encourage research within their own institutions, since leading an industry is preferable to copying others. The collection of new ideas and the testing of their applicability (research) is a component of the pursuit of excellence and can differentiate companies at the top from others in the rear-view mirror.

Financial Knowledge and Business Acumen

"A man with money is no match against a man on a mission."

Doyle Brunson (Pro Poker player)

All companies, businesses, and other entities require resources to carry out their missions. In predominantly financial entities, it is likely that most people who rise to leadership levels are well trained and versed in financial language. The techniques, tools and language are familiar to them, and they feel at home in meetings and conversations which focus on money. And, despite the descriptive terms tax-free, not-for-profit, and charitable trust, the leaders of these structures also need to strive to maximize their resources and realize a 'bottom-line' to fund growth, new programs and payroll increases. But if their mission is not a financial one, the leaders still need to understand the regulations, laws, and functions that provide the background in which they need to operate. In industries such as healthcare, physicians and nurses for example are well known for their lack of education when it comes to financial matters. Some of them don't speak the language and therefore struggle to read and understand financial spreadsheets and statements. They are most comfortable speaking the language of their discipline, the language they learned attending college or while specializing at professional schools as post-graduates. For them, it is vital that they cast their attention beyond their own discipline and learn to operate in the financial world. In finance, experience cannot replace education and weekend business courses, MBAs, and other forms of financial education are highly recommended.

Another area not well understood by leaders not familiar with financial principles is the importance of growth. They know that growth is desirable, but they have not been taught that funding career development of employees, building loyalty, having the resources to continually update equipment, and remaining on the cutting edge of technology all are directly related to growth. They can also miss the link between growth and research funding, also fundamental to competing in almost all industries.

Further, when meetings are being held to discuss financial planning and business strategy, combining this education with doing your homework, is necessary to participate fully and provide leadership, especially when finances are not your core mission. Conversely, attending meetings and proposing ideas that are highly advantageous to your mission, but have no sources of funding, is not viewed as good leadership.

I have witnessed new leaders who sit in meetings where spreadsheets are posted and analyzed but have no idea where to find the information on the spreadsheet and miss the point being made completely. Rather than exposing their lack of knowledge by asking, they sit quietly excluded from the conversation. Asking might take courage and momentary embarrassment, but it would be better than continuing in ignorance. Furthermore, others in the meeting, also not following, would benefit from the ensuing explanation. In short, naivete about financial theory can be harmful to a leader's growth and advance. It is vital that this be prevented by asking and educating oneself in this area. Also, the more senior the leadership role, the more in-depth the financial knowledge needs to be.

Persistence and Perseverance

"Our greatest glory is not in never failing, but in rising up every time we fail." Ralph Waldo Emerson

Many believe that PERSISTENCE is a major requirement for excellent leadership. Certainly, in occasional dynamic situations I have witnessed, being prepared to keep trying no matter how long it takes has resulted in successes that would not have been realized. Giving in strategically is acceptable, never give up. This message conflicts with the idea that doing something that has failed repeatedly and expecting a different outcome, is a form of irrationality. Nevertheless, not giving up is a characteristic that is popular with workers especially when they support the issue being pushed by their leaders.

PERSEVERANCE is slightly different. The saying that "when the going gets tough, the tough gets going", personifies the spirit of perseverance. Workers are asked occasionally to stay late, work through lunch or come in on the weekend, and in the interest of completing a task by a deadline or meeting an emergency need, workers tend to persevere rather than defer. While this cannot be a regular expectation, it is viewed as a sign of dedication and is an attractive characteristic in leaders.

Intimidation

"A culture of intimidation has no justification in any administration"

John Anthony Barrasso. (US Senator, Wyoming)

Anyone who has been in the workplace for a reasonable period will have experienced a measure of intimidation during that time. Unfortunately, it is pervasive in the culture of many entities including businesses, universities, healthcare institutions etc. Leaders, driven themselves by performance goals, are sometimes knowingly passing on this pressure to their team members, and sometimes, unconsciously allow their own anxiety to transmit to those junior to themselves.

Intimidation implies an unhealthy exercise of power that is used to bully or force juniors to work harder or faster or do things against their better judgement. It includes a threat that if this or that goal is not reached, some negative action will follow that will not be welcomed by the junior team members, even extending sometimes to termination. It induces fear, insecurity, and stress and is usually aimed at workers not in a position to counteract or even voice frustration at the perpetrator.

Intimidation of this type might be a component of a generalized culture in an entity or might exist only in isolated sections or under particular leaders. It should also be emphasized that intimidation is not always intended, and leaders are sometimes surprised and even shocked to hear that they are considered intimidating.

It is recognized that intimidation sometimes works for a limited time. Whether because of fear or not, workers labor intensely to satisfy their leaders, and only after a more prolonged time become aware that their lives at work have become unpleasant, and downright threatening. Eventually, workers talk to each other and recognize that their environment has evolved into a punishing grind which they had not initially expected. Ultimately this leads to complaints, frequently expressed to human resource personnel, and some remedy is sought. Conversely it is known that intimidated workers do not give their best, and that better results are accomplished in work environments which are supportive, constructive and respectful. All new leaders should be aware of this issue and should strive to establish a positive work environment.

Authenticity

"Be yourself: everyone else is already taken." Oscar Wilde

Staying true to oneself is one of the most obvious and difficult aspects of leadership. Truth to oneself means that you always act and speak in harmony with your values and ideals. This is difficult because your personal values might well be at odds with those of your entity, leaders or prevailing conditions. However, it is hard to feel good about what you are doing if your actions make you feel guilty, sad, or uncomfortable. All leaders are subject to genuine stress to accomplish their mission, and despite general advice to leave your work at the office, frequently go home searching mentally for solutions that have not been realized at work. While at home or with your family, you should feel free to unwind, separate yourself from work-related stresses and share in the security, safety and joy of family life. When you're not able to be truly AUTHENTIC at work it is very unlikely that you will achieve this at home. At least, you should strive to stay true to yourself in those decisions and actions that you control.

One ideal we should all share is to 'make a difference'. There are two main components to making a difference. One is to make a difference in your mission, (i.e. the products you turn out in your role). If it's the health industry, I'm referring to patients; if it's manufacturing, I'm referring to widgets and so on. The second is to make a difference to your team members, especially so that they too can be true to themselves. By accepting a leadership role, you take on the burden of continually making a difference to those for whom you have been given responsibility. This is an awesome role and making a difference should always be part of the plan for your team.

Another important goal is to continually have the sense that you are engaged in righteous work; and that you are decent, civil, sensitive, kind and considerate. That does not exclude the ability to discipline when appropriate or remedy when things are wrong. It would be incredibly hard to stay true to yourself if you were required to be mean and critical all day long. Feeling good about what you do is of fundamental importance to being true to yourself. Although this is linked directly to your values, there is nothing that will erode your well-being more thoroughly than being engaged in work that you are either ashamed of or fundamentally gives you a sense of guilt. This is true of any work and can be relatively silent in your consciousness until it breaks through and you suddenly realize that what you're doing is contrary to your values. While you might not realize it, inability to sleep well, not smiling much, impatience with loved ones and a lack of interest in socializing are all signs that at work you might not be true to yourself, and you should examine your circumstances and strive to correct your course.

One reason we all work is to earn our keep. To some, money is more important than others. I do not judge this, but I advise against it if you're not thoroughly convinced that you're doing good and that your mission is righteous. I doubt that more money is synonymous with being true to yourself. I doubt that wealth makes people who don't smile, smile more. We are all leaders in some role we play in life. It might be in your family, congregation, sports team, neighborhood or school; but the principles of being true to yourself will apply sometime and will keep stirring your consciousness. As a leader, it is important to recognize that those you lead are also leaders in some other arena and need to be true to themselves too.

Sensitivity

"The real warriors in this world are the ones that see the details of another's soul." Shannon L Alder (author)

SENSITIVITY prevents our differences from dividing us. We have all observed incidents where corporate actions have pleased many but offended or hurt a few. Modern companies and entities are so cosmopolitan and diverse that it is almost impossible to avoid excluding some innocently. I believe it is wiser to intentionally avoid aspects of life that are related to differences. There is a risk that this will result in a sense of reduced fellowship, community and warmth. The remedy is to emphasize and build upon those things that we share and unite us. Some items we all share include a calendar, time, seasons, climate, company mission, diseases, and natural disasters. We live in the USA and share the same calendar. Therefore, we could observe public holidays and celebrations that affect us all and avoid highlighting dates and celebrations not universally shared. An argument could be made for entities that are specifically based on an item that separates us, e.g. a religious school attended exclusively by members of that faith.

Leaders work with employees who earn less than themselves and should be cautious about advising them how and where to spend their resources. What might be a trivial expense to a leader might be beyond the means of some employees.

I have observed a surprising level of insensitivity from leaders when they have, from the podium or by mail, exhorted their employees to make charitable contributions during campaigns for a new building, or a new program. How individuals elect to donate should be private. Leaders should actively support this privacy and should be sensitive about how they approach employees. Sometimes the charities being supported expect relatively more uncommitted income than employees might be able to afford, and it is unfair to put pressure on them, making them feel bad for not donating. Workers should never have to feel guilty for not donating to their place of employment. Simply state that a campaign is currently being initiated and stop there.

I am particularly opposed to leaders contacting employees by personal messages, for example, asking them to fund an amount per mile in a cycling event, when some of those employees might not even be able to afford a bicycle for their own children. This would be insensitive and profoundly unwelcome to employees.

Leaders should nurture an environment of warmth and generosity and leave the decisions regarding donation to individuals. Leaders should remain sensitive to the financial status of their employees and refrain from putting any pressure on them at all.

Another area where sensitivity might be lacking is the assignment of time off from work. While it should be clear that as a leader you are responsible for keeping the entity running smoothly, leaders must recognize the genuine need for workers to have free time off and should institute processes for time off that are as generous as the entity policies allow and provide access and opportunity without interference. Team members should not have to fight for time away from work. The weekends should be time to spend with family or friends completely free of work-related pressures. Not until Monday morning should leaders begin to interact with their team. Sunday evening pressure 'to be ready' for Monday morning is not desirable. Calling people who are out of town on vacation is also not reasonable, so it is important that leaders develop back-up systems which can respond to urgent requirements. These systems should be shared by all team members.

Leaders should not assume or expect that their own work habits will be adopted by team members. A leader who catches up on emails on a weekend day should not expect their team members to be working at the same time. Sending emails on the weekend might create the expectation that the team members must respond on the weekend.

In the unfortunate instance when a team member becomes seriously ill or gets badly injured, leaders share the task of making sure the worker is made to feel valued, respected and supported. Workers do not ask to be sick or hurt, and even if there were doubtful decisions made before an injury, the worker never intended to be unable to work.

Occasionally, insensitivity occurs despite the righteous intent of leaders. Leaders should be aware of this continuously and consider creating a team of multiple level employees who function as guardians of sensitivity. Good leaders are perpetually tuned in to the dignity of their employees and are dedicated to preserving emotional stability and safety.

Conflict, Confrontation and Discipline

"An eye for an eye will only make the whole world blind."

Mahatma Gandhi

Regardless of the type of work you do, and your level of leadership, sporadically you will either be called upon to settle a CONFLICT or become involved in one yourself. Indeed, conflict is a common mechanism for differences of opinion to come to the surface, and it is important to embrace the idea that the greater the variety of opinions on an issue, the richer the resolution will be. Leaders frequently are called upon to resolve disagreements and should expect that conflict resolution will remain part of their daily agenda. The main primary goal of conflict resolution is to turn down the heat and get the differing parties to calm down and engage in forgiveness and compromise. Frequently, conflict is resolved by introducing compromises on each side of the issue and keeping the entity's mission as the prevailing beneficiary.

As a leader you are responsible for recruiting and terminating members of your team. Leaders have to face the possibility of having just completed the building of their ideal team only to be informed by a prominent member that he has been offered a more attractive position, and plans to leave. If the worker is leaving the entity for their new position, it is not unusual for a leader to attempt to reverse the decision to leave. I preferred to ask just once, "is there anything I can do to keep you?". If this elicits a negative response, I ask if there are changes, I could make to avoid this happening to others. I believe that decisions to change positions are complex and once the decision is made there is little to be gained by working to change minds. If the new position a worker is leaving for is inside the same company there are other actions which could be considered, keeping the entity's mission front and center.

When the leader believes a team member is doing more harm than good, he might have to initiate a separation plan. A few principles come to mind. First, the worker's dignity remains of primary importance. Second, no termination or even demotion should be contemplated without making the worker aware of the shortcomings identified and giving the worker an opportunity to remedy them. Third, once the leader is determined to proceed, human resources should be engaged to help with the process. Fourth, wherever possible, the worker's domestic and future well-being should at least be a factor in the timing and conditions of the termination. I would add that, if possible, terminations should be conducted with an HR person present at the time of termination, or directly thereafter. In general leaders should have the ability to have an HR person present in any conversation in which the participants could become highly polarized or angry. This is of course also applicable to situations in which any disciplinary action for a worker is contemplated. There is another point about terminations I should raise.

When a leader in one of your sections indicates they will be leaving, there is a reflex desire to replace that person rapidly, and there is a temptation to appoint the most senior member of the section concerned to be the new leader. This is a word of caution. When you elevate the senior member of the team to be the new leader, they might not have the experience, skill or talent to rapidly fill that spot. You could land up losing the most functional member from the team and have a leader who is not ideal for the leadership position just vacated. The caution is to make sure that this is the best possible person to replace the leader, external or new candidates included, before you take your most functional leader out of the team. This is not a rare scenario and can cripple the performance of that team.

Consistency

"Consistency beats intensity. Consistency beats volume. Consistency beats passion. Consistency dictates results. Consistency is what defines character".

Rich Roll (Author)

Workers soon get to know their leaders; the tone implied by their choice of words and the level of intensity intended by the way ideas are expressed. When a leader suddenly changes this 'style' of communication, workers might view this as inconsistent. Leaders should be careful about sending inconsistent messages to the people they lead. Hearing leaders raise ideas that are one hundred and eighty degrees different from previous statements, is profoundly divisive and intensely disappointing to employees.

We know that circumstances change and that financial pressures might recently exist where none existed before. These conditions would legitimize adopting conflicting policies, but what should not be inconsistent are the values, mission and goals of an organization. Changes in direction should be carefully worded, and previous statements should be reviewed before new policies are released. Employees not in possession of all the information could easily interpret new policies as inconsistent, which could lead to a loss of confidence in leadership.

Once again it behooves leaders to focus on those aspects that they can change and to treat conditions beyond their control differently. It would be destructive to hear employees complaining that last month they said this or that, why did it change so completely just a month later?

CONSISTENCY should be instinctive by the time you rise to a leadership position. Your role and reputation as a leader will be tarnished by allowing inconsistency to typify your communications.

Assistance

"We can't help everyone, but everyone can help someone." Ronald Reagan

There are two basic components to what I have called ASSISTANCE. First and most important is to be willing to seek help when you need it. Sometimes ego can get in the way of admitting that a challenge is too difficult to manage. It might expose a limit in your knowledge or a doubt about your readiness for the job you have.

My experience is that whenever I have sought help, it has enhanced opinions of me by others, and it has always been beneficial in finding a solution to a problem. This does get into the territory of alliances, since it is probable that leaders will develop relationships with a few chosen colleagues that they would feel comfortable approaching for assistance. It is also likely that those you approach for help will also seek advice from you when they come across a difficult issue. This reciprocal sharing of expertise is what makes executive teams most successful and is extremely healthy for the organization. This cooperative partnering is particularly helpful when completely novel challenges arise, such as the Covid pandemic. In this case, there was extensive partnering since nobody had experienced such an event before.

The second component of assistance is making yourself receptive to giving help when asked. It is more likely you will need to give assistance to those who report to you than those on an equal footing. Requests for help should never be brushed off, ignored, or treated lightly. You should be conscious that the requester for help admits that they are struggling and would value your wisdom. Therefore, it is most important that if you are unable to help, you admit it, and assist your employee with finding a solution to the problem. Mentoring is a function of leadership, and this is a perfect example of an opportunity to model cooperative partnering to them. Refusing to help would be wrong but encouraging an employee to do their own research and discovery might be valuable, particularly when you are trying to build confidence in someone. This would be a judgement call, and one of the reasons you are now a leader.

Follow-up

"Leadership is about three-fourths show-the-way and about one-fourth follow-up." James E. Faust

Even though you expect your team to carry out your policies, there is no skill more important than routine intentional FOLLOW-UP. It is just a fact of life that when no follow-up is expected, items slip from the list and delays ensue. Follow-up is not an inborn or reflex action. It is an action that is necessary, does not imply distrust, and is fundamental to continual success. Leaders must be able to balance follow-up with micromanagement. Some will interpret too much follow-up as a leader trying to over-manage them.

Once members of the team get used to follow-up calls and actions, they come to expect them, and they perform accordingly. Conversely, it is embarrassing for leaders to have to tell their bosses that a deadline was missed, or some action has not yet been approached. This item is related to the section on punctuality. You do not want to be identified as the cause of even one late action, never mind repeated delays.

In a related thought, repeated delays are an alert that the employee is not up to the task or is chronically overloaded. No one wants to fail. There are multiple reasons for being chronically late, and it is the burden of leaders to dig into why this is happening. It is important to eliminate other causes of delays before concluding that a team member is unable to cope and might need help or a replacement.

Regardless, some measure of follow-up should be a leader's work habit. There is no reason not to.

Punctuality

"Arriving late is a way of saying your own time is more valuable than the time of the person who waited for you." Karen Joy Fowler (Author)

Being on time is important in two senses. One is being on time for live meetings, appointments, and timed engagements. The other is about delivering services, communications, goods and promises when you indicated you would.

Even though occasionally being late for a meeting may be unavoidable, being late regularly is poor form. I have frequently observed the main advocate for this or that item on an agenda arrive in the meeting after the item has been discussed and put to a vote by Robert's Rules. The latecomer proceeds to reopen the matter despite the decision being decided already by a vote of the attendees. Now, as I indicated, if this happens very occasionally, it is irritating. If it happens frequently, it is intolerable, and the reputation of the latecomer will be rapidly destroyed. I have seen senior team members lose their positions over this issue. If you are running late for a meeting and you are a key participant for the agenda item you might miss, you should call in ahead and indicate your regrets and ask for the item to be delayed. You should also always excuse yourself for being late when you ultimately arrive. Once a leader is identified as "always being late", their credibility is compromised.

Other team members begin not to take them seriously, and their opportunities and ability to persuade others of the value of their agendas is undermined. Soon, they become the subject of derision and humor and intentionally isolate themselves among those whose support is most critical to their success.

Similarly, if one is regularly late in turning in work products, the system cannot wait. Once again, communicating delay for completion is critical, but if this is a regular occurrence, there is little that will reverse the negative impact of chronic tardiness. Initially, your late delivery will cause raised eyebrows, but if recurrent, team members will be reluctant to entrust important work to you and eventually will cease to do so. It is not possible to convince hard-working people that your tardiness is acceptable when others are on time. Your ability to persuade others and to influence people (key requirements for leadership) will be harmed irreversibly.

Homework

"By failing to prepare, you're preparing to fail." Benjamin Franklin

When we were in school, we yearned for the days when HOMEWORK would not be an expectation. I have been lucky to have been taught by a previous mentor that homework never ends. In the past, good texts on performance in the workplace have focused on how meetings are not productive or valuable in many instances. My own experience is that meetings among leaders sometimes tend to be entertainment sessions, where the chair of the meeting prepares and circulates an agenda, and the participants leading each agenda item present the issues. The rest of the attendees tend to come into the meeting without preparing, reading or doing any research to make themselves familiar with the material announced in the circulated agenda. In essence, they expect the material to be set before them, like a plate at mealtimes, and they expect to listen (if interested), analyze (if they listened), and vote if a decision needs to be made.

The quickest way to differentiate yourself as a leader is to do the homework. Research the material circulated in advance, gather your own thoughts on the topic, and be ready to comment critically on the merits and value of the proposals. Frequently, you will be the only one with a vote in the room who fully understands the ramifications of the decision that might be made. You will have an opportunity to give your opinion based on knowledge and persuade or influence others in the direction you believe would best benefit the attendees at the meeting. That is leadership. Without the homework, you are just being entertained.

Unfortunately, our individual lives are so busy, so packed with items of concern, that we are too distracted or weary to take the time needed to do our homework. The person leading the item on the agenda has researched their agenda items well and is usually presenting them because they are passionate about the next steps to be taken. This might be an advantage to the group he or she represents (possibly selfishly). To bring a balanced view on concerns brought to a committee meeting, others in the meeting need to consider the pros and cons rationally. This cannot take place during the meeting alone, it requires research, education, and focused thought – i.e. homework!

If the same attendee is the only person who regularly does their homework and is the only person regularly raising a reasonable alternate view to the presenter, that person will be regarded as smarter than most and will build their reputation as a leader. The need for homework never expires.

Discretion

"Judgement is not upon all occasions required, but discretion always is." Lord Chesterfield (Philip Dormer Stanhope, 4th Earl of Chesterfield 1694 – 1773)

In politics, it appears that leaking information is almost expected. In professional and industrial entities, leaking confidential information shared in leadership meetings is highly problematic. As a leader, you are frequently a party to sensitive information which could possibly be harmful if it was known outside the confines of the leadership team. It could harm your entity, individual careers, and strategic plans that have been discussed on the committee. When committees have these private discussions, it is understood by attendees that the information shared there is private, but at some other time, in conversations and even socially, DISCRETE information can be discussed without even realizing how a previous meeting's privacy is being breached.

Leaders should be aware of this possibility, and especially because when the information is out, it is often obvious where the leak occurred. Discretion is close to honesty. It is presumed that by the time you have risen in rank to be discussing important private issues that you understand the importance of discretion. Once it is recognized that the leak came from you, your chances of being entrusted with discrete material again are compromised. As in rescuing honesty, rescuing discretion is challenging. Team members will be guarded about openly discussing private matters in your presence, and your ability to lead will be impaired.

I should mention that when absolute discretion is applied, some outsiders who knew the meeting would occur might feel excluded if no aspects of the meeting are shared after the conclusion of the meeting. Leaders should consider indicating what is discreet and what can be shared.

Routine Administrative Busy Work

"We are what we repeatedly do. Excellence, then, is not an act, but a habit." Aristotle

Unfortunately, all jobs have duties to perform which are less exciting and difficult to sustain. I refer to these tasks as ROUTINE ADMINISTRATIVE BUSY WORK. However, delayed completion of these tasks leads to a domino effect, where downstream work does not get done until the routine task is moved to the next step. If one is managing this next step and the person delaying the progress of the task turns out to be the same person repeatedly, a narrative is set up which rapidly snowballs into a 'reputation'. The delaying worker gains a record as a person who holds up productivity, and the next step is even more damaging - workers begin to suggest that that person should be omitted from the process.

Therefore, I am suggesting that leaders must have the discipline and commitment to complete routine work with punctuality and never be identified as 'holding things up'. Even when that work is boring or not identified as important, leaders should avoid being the bottleneck. This advice has the potential to conflict with my comments warning leaders to do their homework, and not to act or without adequate review and understanding. Acting impulsively will frequently come back to haunt leaders who never gave the matter enough thought or without doing some homework.

Another area where conflict might arise is with other advice I will give about "following your discomfort". If there is routine busy work that somehow makes you uncomfortable, you have a responsibility to hesitate and dig deeper into the process. If your instincts are telling you to hold up, something is being presented that reminds you of a previous experience and alerts you to dwell a bit longer and investigate what is bothering you.

Routine busy work impacts all levels of leadership. Even junior workers can easily identify work they would rather not do and might believe is a waste of time. This work is called many things. 'Scutwork' is a frequently used term for this dreary duty. Nevertheless, my advice is to get it done before deadlines expire. Once you recognize that you ae reluctant to complete this type of work, you should discipline yourself to put time aside during work hours to complete these tasks.

Pondering

"The key to great learning is understanding a little at a time."
John Locke (English philosopher 1632 – 1704)

This section could also be called ruminating, thinking or even meditating. It is about spending calm time churning issues that have occurred recently, how you could have managed them differently or better, and considering solutions to challenges that are still ahead of you. The bad side of PONDERING is that it could become stressful or even obsessive.

I would guess that most leaders ponder to some extent or another, and that their families might say they are spending good family time bringing the office into their homes. Nevertheless, I believe that ponderers are exercising their dedication to their careers and need this time to come up with new ideas or settle with previous decisions they have opposed. Therefore, I believe that pondering is not only healthy but necessary for some leaders. Indeed, it is possible that just as spiritual leaders recommend meditation, so leaders should be encouraged to take the time to ponder if they need it. Similarly, families should be encouraged to grant their members who are leaders the freedom to ponder and even encourage it, if it seems fitting.

It is just as important to avoid pondering becoming purely stressful or obsessive. This is delicate material since the transition could be subtle and a cause for disagreement within families. We should encourage open dialogue about these issues and avoid being prescriptive. Nevertheless, some would insist that pondering is as important as doing the work, and leaders should feel free to do it when needed.

Follow Your Discomfort

"Intuition is a very powerful thing, more powerful than intellect, in my opinion." Steve Jobs

This is not an original thought, but I have experience where my discomfort with a recruit helped me avoid making an error. I believe thoroughly that 'instinct' is more about memory and experience than prescience. Feeling uncomfortable with an idea, a policy, or task, is your subconscious alerting you that something feels wrong about this and that you have faced a related decision before with which you were not pleased. So, my advice is that you should not ignore that uncomfortable 'nudge' that you are experiencing and temporarily pause while you reconsider. In the case I mentioned above, I delayed committing to a very attractive recruit based on DISCOMFORT which later proved to be a wise decision.

Luckily, I have observed my leaders exercising this advice. Frequently, the proposal is met with a quizzical look or silence when some acknowledgement is expected. That is a clue to go back and review the idea. It might still be a good idea, but it might not fit because there are conditions about which you are naive.

Regardless of the origin of the discomfort, my advice is to pause and reconsider. It is an alert to do more homework or seek advice from another leader who might or might not share your concern. This would be an example of a valuable delay and should not be included in your routine administrative busy work. If something feels uncomfortable, it might well be your honesty at work. When there is even a hint of dishonesty about an intended action, always follow your discomfort by reconsideration or seeking another opinion. Honesty is the most valuable currency in the business of leadership, and your comfort with a proposed action should always be as solid as a solvent bank account.

Vengeance

"Vengeance is the act of turning anger in on yourself. On the surface it may be directed at someone else, but it is a surefire recipe for arresting emotional recovery." Jane Goldman (Born 1970. Screenwriter, producer)

There is no denying that being in a leadership position gives one power over others. Using that power to punish individuals who have annoyed you, opposed you or voted against your proposals is simply an abuse of power. Any sign of that behavior is an alert that the leader is unfit for a leadership position.

Is the above paragraph generally accepted as correct? Not necessarily. Some believe revenge is a part of leadership. Some seek leadership to take revenge. I have observed vengeance seeking among leaders and have found it to be abhorrent. When it happens, it focuses on the narcissistic side of people and underscores the insecurity of the offending leader. Authentic leaders welcome all opinions, contrary and supportive, and recognize how multiple opinions enrich the final answer you arrive at. In the same vein, true balance can only be achieved if both sides of an issue are aired and weighed. In so much as balance is perceived as good, contrary opinions should be welcomed, if not actively recruited, and should never be a reason to punish. I have seen leaders who have used power to punish, end up dying on the same sword they wielded and never understand why. The phrase ‘being hoisted on your own petard’ elegantly describes that outcome.

This is one of those aspects of leadership that should not need to be mentioned in this type of text. Leaders should instinctively know that this is poor conduct. I mention it here because of the rare exceptions. A good way to understand and avoid vengeance is to focus on the corollary, which is humility. Advice to remain humble in your actions is perhaps better advice than avoiding vengeance.

Humor

"A sense of humor is part of the art of leadership.... of getting things done." Dwight D. Eisenhower

While HUMOR is not a requirement of good leadership, its total absence will be noticed and missed. It is not necessary to tell jokes, since this might come across as trivial or undermine the tone you require at any given point. But when a humorous incident or image comes to mind, it can be raised to humanize and lighten a serious moment. It is also welcomed by employees and will be perceived as warm and friendly.

A total lack of humor is fine for many interactions but misses opportunities for stress relief and changes in pace. People might not notice a lack of humor for a while but will eventually know that you are always serious and will register that you take yourself too seriously in the long term. There is a risk that employees or team members might not like you as much if you never display a smile or laugh. Leadership is not a popularity contest, so this is not that much of a risk, but there is an opportunity with a humorous break, to appear to be human and real and should be seized if available.

If you find a moment or instance funny, make sure it doesn't embarrass a member of the team when you raise it. Team members with a good sense of humor will roll with it, but those who are less secure might be offended. Poking fun at yourself is always safer and usually welcomed. But I would advise strongly against making fun of others, especially juniors. This would surely erode trust and respect.

This too is a subject which, in most individuals reaching leadership positions, should not be needed. It is mentioned because physiognomy continually devoid of humor, is tiring and discouraging.

Appreciation, Celebration and Reward

"None of us is as smart as all of us." Ken Blanchard (Author)

Leaders should know that praise for their team members is like water to a plant. For the sake of completeness, I mention here how important it is for leaders to vocally deliver words of APPRECIATION whenever possible. If you keep repeating appreciative messages, they will be heard, and in turn, greatly appreciated.

Similarly, celebrating successes and awards is very meaningful. All employees want to do well and please their bosses, and noticing their achievements makes it all worthwhile. Celebrations for success can range from a simple thank you or card to a local gathering with the team. Certifications which demanded hard work and extensive preparation should be celebrated with as big a group as funds allow. They do not occur often and contribute directly to the success of the entity.

If the company is lucky enough to earn competitive awards, these should be widely recognized and celebrated. Awards are rare and can be used to publicly advertise the entity, especially in competition with local companies in the same market.

Regardless of certifications and awards, it is simple to say thank you whenever possible and should become habitual for leaders when interacting with their teams.

Dress code

"People react well to a person they like the looks of." Mary Quant

Time has certainly altered dress codes for in-office employees. Employees working at home and attending computer meetings should be dressed as if they were in the office. Over time, dress codes have become less formal, and simultaneously, less likely to be controversial or an issue to cause strife in a company. Despite the general acceptance of suits or sports coats without ties, I prefer a more conservative approach. You might have noticed that CEOs, Presidents, and Chief executives in general still wear suits with ties, and women still wear slacksuits with blouses or business suits with a skirt and jacket. Some companies have endorsed and accepted Fridays as informal days, but if senior meetings are scheduled, senior executives will still be formally dressed. Senior executives apart, sports coats with no tie remain the standard for men and slack suits for women.

If for any reason, external representatives are in the office, I would tend to advise leaders to wear more formal dress. No one ever was criticized for dressing too well. When leaders dress in a suit and tie, they tend to command respect more readily. In some professions, suits and ties are expected. In others, less formal dress is very acceptable.

In general, work attire is dictated by the nature of your work and company policy. I would advise a liberal approach to work attire unless you're in a hospital or a site where more formal attire is the tradition (e.g. courts of law). Many companies object to uncovered tattoos although those too have become more acceptable. Untidy hair and wild make up and nails still raise objections even though I have never observed that type of thing negatively impact work. Once again, I personally advise more formal dress than is popular or accepted.

Education

"For the best return on your money, pour your purse into your head." Benjamin Franklin

Although executive teams are composed of a broad variety of individuals, with a full array of educational qualifications, by the time they are elevated to leadership roles, they are focused on those departments assigned to them by their leadership. The broader the educational experience on a team, the richer the experience will be at the executive table. But it is likely that they are, in many instances, leading departments or programs quite distinct from their formal EDUCATION. Their credibility depends in part on their willingness to defer to expertise, and in part to their rigor in learning about the discipline they are leading.

Leaders have a duty to raise their own education about areas beyond their own sphere of expertise. This responsibility can be accomplished in a variety of formats and experiences but should be achieved by a sense of personal duty and desire for self-improvement rather than by instruction from bosses. True, once you are in the workforce and in a leadership position, there will no longer be tests or examinations, but your performance in areas where you are not formally educated will quickly be judged by smart team members if decisions are based on naivete or ignorance.

Since there are no tests or examinations, once you accept a

leadership role in a particular area, only you will know when your basic knowledge is weak. This should immediately create two tasks. One is to identify experienced, knowledgeable team members and build relationships with them to obtain advice and to build trust that you are keen to learn and appreciate their help. It is also advisable to establish this kind of relationship with other executive team members who might in a past position have had responsibility for an area you now have been assigned. They could be a good source of advice to you. Second is to identify courses, reading material and sources of current and new literature so that you can privately build your own confidence.

If you have been promoted to a leadership position based on the expertise you have acquired either through formal EDUCATION or experience, you should make sure you stay up to date in that area. It is enormously advantageous to be considered an expert in an area important to the mission of your company. Similarly, if your own industry or research has led to you having a gimmick or shortcut to a goal, this too is an asset to your employer, and you should make sure this is known to your bosses and that you make it available whenever appropriate.

Related to education is a further piece of advice about getting your own ego in the way of getting help when you need it. If you come up with an idea that is new or different, you should test it with colleagues you trust and avoid even a hint of resistance to their thoughts in areas with which you are still relatively unfamiliar. Make sure you do not stay committed to a potentially unsuccessful path. You must strive to be viewed as open and flexible; while sustaining the reputation you have built for creativity and innovation.

Friends, Alliances and Relationships

"Outside of a dog, a book is a man's best friend. Inside it is too dark to read." Groucho Marx

Any leader will know how important it is to work on relationships. Common sense teaches us that when we need help to achieve any challenging task, our relationships make the difference. However, this section is more subtle than that. I will discuss friendships first.

FRIENDS you have made at work along the road to success should remain close friends of yours despite the possibility that they might not have advanced as rapidly as you and might now report to you or a colleague with whom you are closely associated. This raises the possibility that you might have to change the way you relate to friends at work, or you might even have to criticize, discipline or impact that friend's job security. Can this friend remain as close to you as before? Would you act the same if this employee wasn't your friend? It depends on your friendship and your past interactions. Sometimes, it's best to distance yourself from such friendships to avoid appearing biased. This matter could also affect future friendships and might influence your interactions with new acquaintances. I have had friends I was able to sustain as before, and I have had some I decided to change. I have also decided in the past to step back from social interactions with people to whom I report out of a need to be sensitive to the possibility that I might place them in a difficult position. In my experience, there is no perfect solution to this issue. It must be sorted out as you go. It is important to know about it and to be prepared to adjust if necessary.

Alliances are different, in that they do not necessarily require warmth between you. Alliances are when you recognize that another individual might be able to make you more successful, and you intentionally build a relationship with them. Is this using people? If your intent is to make alliances mutually beneficial, I do not believe so. You can help each other! But if you pursue an alliance for a selfish advantage and drop that alliance once it is completed, it is exploiting them. Once again, there is no obvious advice which applies in all cases. If your intent is to take advantage of them, it is dishonest and should be avoided. If you just go with the flow and end up recognizing an opportunity to benefit from a connection, it is better to state up front what your purpose is. It might still develop into a mutually beneficial relationship. Being aware of the challenges is most important, and you will work out your own approach as you advance in leadership. Always remember that the other person probably recognizes this too.

There are also strategic alliances. For example, if you are in the business of making food, it would be important to develop contacts and trustworthy connections in the farming industry. This theory applies across the board in business, and these relationships sometimes take years to build. Similarly, there are tactical aspects as to how to talk to people in the farming industry versus the insurance industry or the clothing industry. It is incumbent on leaders to learn and develop the skills to nurture respectful and productive relationships with leaders and important stakeholders in industries related to their own. Hospital executives must know how to interact with physicians, and automobile dealers must learn how to relate to parts manufacturers and so on. Whereas patients are the main customers of hospitals, physicians are also customers. The interactions of leaders related or connected to your industry are vitally important too and should not be disrespected or ignored.

Strategy

"Without strategy, execution is aimless. Without execution, strategy is useless." Morris Chang

At various levels of leadership, you will find yourself in small group meetings or a range of one-on-one meetings where it is important for you to be able to read body language, understand posturing and have insight into what other participants really intend to gain from the dialogue. So often leaders do not say exactly what they want while they're busy evaluating what they think you want. You might be meeting with external leaders who are competing with you at some level, or you might be in an internal meeting where leaders of other departments in your institution are competing with you for budgetary support. Either way the ability to understand the true intent of your co-attendees is critically important to how you develop your own STRATEGY going forward.

Some leaders you'll meet are better than others at sorting out each attendee's unstated goals, or discerning between posturing, aiming high or just stating their aims. Reading body language is a combination of experience, common sense, business acumen and observation. Also, it requires a measure of modesty, since it is important to be open to the idea that you might just be wrong and could make mistakes based on your erroneous evaluations. Regardless, you should get used to asking yourself what the other participants really want. Can you discern their strategy? Good deals are made when both sides of an agreement leave the table feeling that they got enough of what they originally wanted to advance their own agenda. You can frequently sense when that state has been reached, and if not, it is a skill you should master. One of the most crucial steps in negotiating successfully is a reasonably accurate understanding of where your opposition wants to be.

To many leaders this talent is inbred or acquired subconsciously along the way, but if you feel you don't yet have it, you must increase the sensitivity of your own antenna until you grow confident that you are reading the table well. Once you do, you will be able to attend meetings and listen more than you speak with a view to being less transparent yourself. I would rather others are sitting wondering what you really are looking for, than them confidently pushing you to your limit because they knew all along where that was. This talent is not unlike playing poker with a group of poker players who are as good as you are. It's ok to bluff occasionally but it is better to have good cards in your hand when you bet.

Another component of this skill is to have a thorough knowledge of the facts about the subject you are discussing. This brings us to doing your homework. You cannot expect to be successful regularly in negotiations or debates, if you don't have background information at your fingertips. Your strategy should be based on knowledge rather than guess work. It is incumbent upon the leader to make sure he has gained all discoverable information in preparing for meetings. Therefore, it behooves you to research and study the angles and history of each situation in which you plan to participate, and especially if you plan to come to an agreement.

Once you are successfully making these judgements, your confidence in attending these meetings will increase, anxiety will be manageable, and you will be respected by others who attend. Reading body language and reading between the lines contribute to all the material you use to clarify your strategy. As you mature, gain experience and knowledge, your reputation at the negotiating table will grow and success will follow. You have to learn faster than the environment is changing.

Managing Your Ego: The Rumor Mill

"Words spoken can never be recalled." Wentworth Dillon (Earl of Roscommon. 1637 - 1685)

The moment you accept a new position in leadership; you take on a new number of employees who report to you either directly or indirectly. The new reports will watch their leader closely, and a narrative will form based on their observations. If this offends you, leadership is not for you. It is perfectly natural for this to happen and is frequently based on the earliest observations made. The 'RUMOR MILL' will have proponents and opponents contributing to the narrative, and the earlier it is formed, the more likely it is that it will be premature, inaccurate and unreliable. As a leader you should realize that gossip is expected and you should not be stressed, obsessed or fixated on what they're saying.

On the other hand, it is always wise to keep your ear close to the ground. While the Rumor Mill is often based on superficial and false information, it is nevertheless a prevailing opinion, and it is an indication or signal of how you are perceived. To the extent there are aspects of your reputation that are negative and could be remedied, the only way to approach them is if you know about them. Also, you would create an opportunity to discover what you do well and what you could build upon to enhance your performance even more.

There are tests and feedback programs that can give you a good idea on a limited range of behaviors, and if you hired a coach to help develop your leadership skills, they would certainly want you to ask some of your reports to complete carefully constructed questionnaires which can give you clues as to your strengths and weaknesses. But once again, I would not recommend a slavish belief in what these tests show, I have known them to be quite contrary to my opinion of other individuals.

Regardless, the Rumor Mill will persist, and you should not be overly concerned about what people say. In the long run, if you do the right thing, spread warmth and kindness, and bring consistency to your team, they will support you much more intensely than you expect, or than the rumor mill might predict.

Timing

"Observe due measure, for right timing is in all things the most important factor." Hesiod (776 BC. Greek poet)

While the 'soonest possible' is a good approach, I am compelled to caution the new leader that TIMING can be crucial in conducting good leadership. Many years ago, I learned about the inexorable pressure that the ticking clock might bring. I was discussing the pros and cons of buying futures on the stock market and was educated about how important the clock is when it comes to paying for your stock. The intent is to buy low and bet that in a certain amount of time the stock will be worth much more, and you could just collect the positive difference – profit. But what if the stock begins to sag in value, and you're looking at the best time to sell, not knowing when or if the stock will recover or grow in value. As the clock ticks your money is dwindling, but it might recover! In time or not?

In leadership timing is also most important. In making decisions about resources, supplies, volumes, turnover, and value the clock can make the difference between a good decision and a disaster. Factors such as regulations, tariffs, weather, politics and competition, to name a few, can tilt a decision about manufacturing deadlines, price predictions and prompt delivery. Supply and demand are complex matters, and we cannot predict the future. Furthermore, penalties are frequently built into expectations on the ground, and being too late can be a disastrous outcome.

Sometimes your opponent across the table or even your partner might have knowledge not in the open, that can have a serious impact on your ability to meet a promise. Perhaps you feel pressured in a negotiation and in your ignorance, you embrace or deny an advantage that turns into the opposite when you discover the reality of timing later.

As stated above, there is no viewing the future, and errors will happen. In this format, the best advice is to always think about the twists and turns of the ticking clock. The size risks you take are linked to the victories you win, but without due regard to the possibility of timing anomalies, your risk might exceed the advantage you fail to gain.

Silence

"Better to remain silent and be thought a fool than to speak out and remove all doubt." Abraham Lincoln

I mention in two other locations in this book how if you want to be truly articulate you must know when not to speak. Since SILENCE is such a powerful arrow in your quiver, I raise it again. The quote above is wisdom at its best. There are multiple reasons why staying silent is so important.

Another phrase comes to mind in this discussion. You were given two ears and one mouth so that you will listen more and talk less. When you don't speak it often says more than when you do. I did point out that when approaching a senior with an idea, a silent response is them hinting that the idea will not fly for some reason or another. The same applies to you when a junior approaches you with an idea that does not gel with your current plan.

Similarly, when at the negotiating table silence is potentially a considerable advantage. If you imagine you're at a negotiating table and your opponent suddenly raises a point not previously on the record. Not responding to it leaves your opponent in a difficult situation. He or she does not know whether you are outright rejecting it, whether it is so trivial you don't care, whether you didn't notice it or any other possibility. In the meantime, you can't tell if this is vital to your opponent yet. You want time to ponder the consequences, bring it back to your team, or use it later to gain some other edge. So, you wait. This is a case of silence giving you time to process the addition of a new request and broaden your understanding of what your opponent holds as important, i.e. time for reflection.

If the situation you're in is testy and conflict is building, staying silent might prevent further escalation and allow emotions to calm while you process what has raised the stakes. If you answer in anger, you might drive the tension higher and say something regrettable that might impair your success later. This is a form of protection for you, using patience and caution rather than reaction. Furthermore, a silent response during a disagreement can put pressure on other participants to speak and perhaps uncover something you had missed, revealing an unknown point that might have fooled you otherwise.

This discussion makes it obvious how important using silence can be. It also helps you manage silence when you are confronted by it. It will set off a thought process which alerts you to tread carefully and be patient. Sometimes if you perceive that someone is using silence to gain an advantage the timing might be appropriate to try another approach on the same topic, thereby pressuring your opponent to comment even if they passed on the first opportunity.

It is not possible to predict all circumstances in which silence would be a better choice than reacting, but silence is frequently a good choice and can facilitate clarity while you consider your options.

Things to Avoid:

1. The 'new Sheriff in town" approach. When you take over a new assignment, be gentle about the changes you make until you fully understand the full consequences of those changes. For big changes, it is wise to wait until the new team has got to know you. You cannot assume that everything about previous processes was bad.

2. Avoid 'reinventing the wheel'. Once something has failed it is futile to go back there. Even if you change only parts of a process, frame it as new. Workers are loathe to repeat past errors.

3. It is not collaborative to flat ignore suggestions and new ideas.

4. Sticking to a highly criticized or unpopular policy or process is unlikely to be successful.

5. Remember the admonition that to keep doing the same thing and expecting a different outcome is regarded as 'insanity'.

6. Do not narrow down your friendships and allegiances to an obvious 'in-group'. Those outside the group will resent this

enormously and strongly oppose any action you take.

7. Shy away from appearing fearful of highly intense, risky or aggressive proposals. Your team wants to see you be strong and represent them assertively.

8. Even when an idea sounds 'crazy' to you, never turn it down flat on the first pass. Reserve your right to explore and research the idea.

9. If as a leader you are forced to take a stand on an issue at odds with your team's opinion or preference, you need to explain why you're making the decision. You cannot just leave them in the dark. Don't put your superiors under the bus. You could refer to new circumstances that you're not yet allowed to share as the reason. If you do not explain yourself somewhat, trust becomes a risk.

10. As a leader you have the freedom to take time off when you desire. This is a caution not to exceed reasonable time away from work, or to be unavailable when you are at work. It is reasonable to delegate someone to be available when you are away, but ultimately your responsibility does not go away because you were absent. A leader cannot lead effectively

when they are absent.

11. Even though you might have good cause, never walk out. You cannot impact on anything when you are not there. You might think at the time that the best message you can deliver is to opt out, but this eliminates you from the immediate next steps. If the environment is so toxic, you can't stay, rather than walk out, suggest taking a break, or suspending the conversation until all have cooled down.

12. You might be pressured one day to face a group of team members who have complaints. Take them one at a time. My advice is to never hold a complaints meeting; it might put you in the minority against a hostile group and unless you have all the answers you will not be happy with the outcome

.

13. Whenever you have the idea that a requested meeting might be about human resource issues, elect to have a third-party present. You could state up front that you have asked to have your employee of choice to be present to ensure fairness.

Positive leadership words

Accountability	Advise
Analyze	Appreciate
Ask	Be present
Be sensitive	Bring out the best
Care	Challenge
Collaborate	Compliment
Communication	Decide
Encourage	Energize
Evaluate	Guide
Humor	Inform
Lead	Listen
Motivate	Organize
Praise	Predict
Promote	Reassign
Recognizing	Relationships
Respect	Set Standards
Trust	Warmth

I'd love to hear from you!

I value your thoughts and feedback on this book. Please feel free to share your reflections, suggestions, or experiences by writing to me at: **braesleader@gmail.com**

www.ingramcontent.com/pod-product-compliance
Lightning Source LLC
LaVergne TN
LVHW051044210926
848486LV00001B/12